HOW TO MAKE NATURAL LIQUID AND SOLID PERFUMES

DR MIRIAM KINAI

CONTENTS

ACKNOWLEDGMENTS

I would like to express my sincere gratitude to everyone who contributed in one way or another to the development of this publication.

I would especially like to thank http://www.zazzle.com/ChristianArtGifts for their photographs.

1

HOW TO BLEND NATURAL FRAGRANCES

Essential oils are natural fragrances that can be used to make organic liquid and solid perfumes.

To create a well balanced natural perfume, you have to consider the volatility of the different essential oils so that you can mix them appropriately.

To do this, you have to know whether an essential oil is a top note, a **middle note or a base note.**

***

Top Notes

These are the essential oils with scents that evaporate the fastest and therefore they are the first ones you smell. These scents are generally light, flowery, fruity and uplifting.

Examples of top notes include bergamot essential oil, clary sage essential oil, eucalyptus essential oil, lemon essential oil, orange essential oil, petitgrain essential oil and tea tree essential oil.

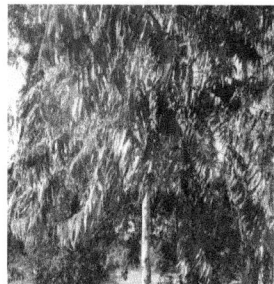 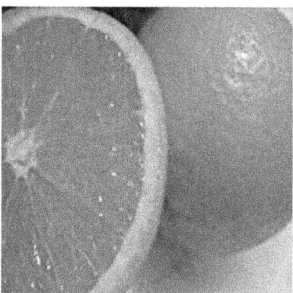 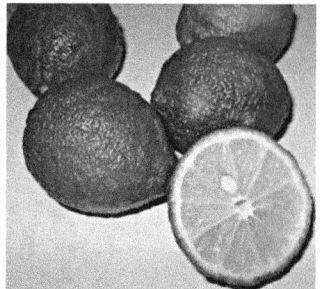

***

Middles Notes

These scents do not evaporate as fast as the top notes. They are generally spicy, herbal and balancing.

Examples of middle notes include Roman and German chamomile essential oil, cypress essential oil, geranium essential oil, juniper berry essential oil, lavender essential oil, sweet marjoram essential oil, peppermint essential oil, rosemary essential oil and rosewood essential oil.

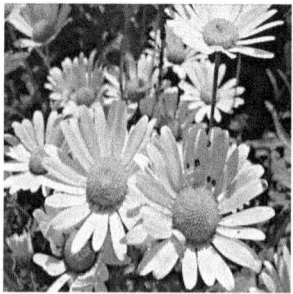 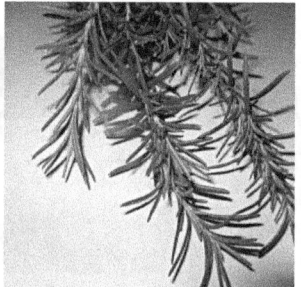 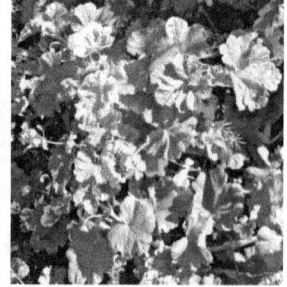

Base Notes

These scents are the slowest to evaporate and therefore the last ones you smell. They are generally heavy and woodsy.

Examples of base notes include cedarwood essential oil, clove essential oil, ginger essential oil, helichrysum essential oil, jasmine essential oil, neroli essential oil, patchouli essential oil, rose essential oil, sandalwood essential oil, vanilla essential oil and ylang ylang essential oil.

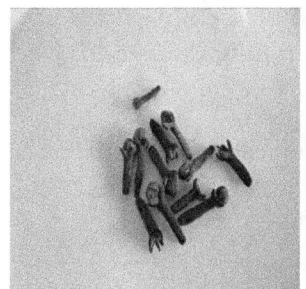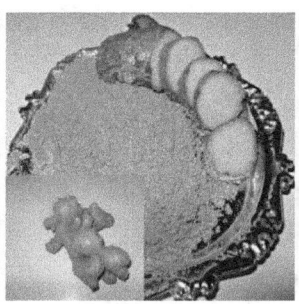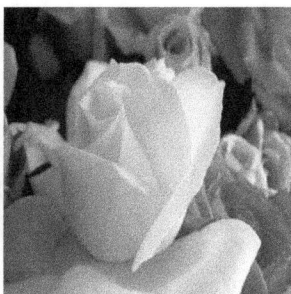

*****

General Rules for Blending Essential Oils

1. Decide what condition you want your essential oil blend to manage.

2. Choose approximately 3 essential oils that can manage that condition.

3. Divide those essential oils into top notes, middle notes and base notes.

4. Blend your essential oils by adding 1 drop of the base note for every 2 drops of the middle note and 3 drops of the top note into a dark bottle.

5. Begin by adding the base notes and after adding each essential oil into the bottle, swirl it around and smell it before you add the next essential oil.

6. After getting a scent that pleases you, you can now add the essential oils blend to the other ingredients of your natural perfume.

7. Always have a notebook at hand to record the number of drops of each essential oil you have added to create that particular blend.

***

Practical Example 1 of Blending Essential Oils

1. Decide what condition you want your perfume essential oil blend to manage.

Stress

2. Choose approximately three essential oils that can manage that condition.

Essential oils that are used to manage stress include lavender, Roman chamomile, bergamot, clary sage, petitgrain, geranium, marjoram, peppermint, rose, sandalwood and ylang ylang essential oils

Chosen essential oils: Lavender essential oil, clary sage essential oil and ylang ylang essential oil

3. Divide those essential oils into top notes, middle notes and base notes.

Top note: clary sage, Middle note: lavender, Base note: ylang ylang

4. Blend your essential oils by adding 1 drop of the base note for every 2 drops of the middle note and 3 drops of the top note into a dark bottle.

5. Begin by adding the base notes and after adding each essential oil into the bottle, swirl it around and smell it before you add the next essential oil.

a) Put 1 drop of ylang ylang essential oil in a dark bottle, swirl and sniff

b) Add 2 drops of lavender essential oil, swirl and sniff

c) Add 3 drops of clary sage essential oil, swirl and sniff

6. After getting a scent that pleases you, add the essential oil blend to the other natural perfume ingredients.

***

Practical Example 2 of Blending Essential Oils

1. Decide what condition you want your perfume essential oil blend to manage.

Sadness or Depression

2. Choose approximately three essential oils that can manage that condition.

Essential oils used to treat depression include bergamot, clary sage, Roman chamomile, lavender, rosemary, rose and ylang ylang essential oil.

Chosen essential oils: Rosemary essential oil, bergamot essential oil and ylang ylang essential oil

3. Divide those essential oils into top notes, middle notes and base notes.

Top note: bergamot, Middle note: rosemary, Base note: ylang ylang

4. Blend your essential oils by adding 1 drop of the base note for every 2 drops of the middle note and 3 drops of the top note into a dark bottle.

5. Begin by adding the base notes and after adding each essential oil into the bottle, swirl it around and smell it before you add the next essential oil.

a) Put 1 drop of ylang ylang essential oil in a dark bottle, swirl and sniff

b) Add 2 drops of rosemary essential oil, swirl and sniff

c) Add 3 drops of bergamot essential oil, swirl and sniff

6. After getting a scent that pleases you, add the essential oil blend to the other natural perfume ingredients.

Practical Example 3 of Blending Essential Oils

1. Decide what condition you want your essential oil blend to manage.

Excessive Anger

2. Choose approximately three essential oils that can manage that condition.

Essential oils that are used for anger management include bergamot, clary sage, orange, petitgrain, Roman chamomile, lavender, rose and ylang ylang essential oil.

Chosen essential oils: Lavender essential oil, orange essential oil and ylang ylang essential oil

3. Divide those essential oils into top notes, middle notes and base notes.

Top note: orange, Middle note: lavender, Base note: ylang ylang

4. Blend your essential oils by adding 1 drop of the base note for every 2 drops of the middle note and 3 drops of the top note into a dark bottle.

5. Begin by adding the base notes and after adding each essential oil into the bottle, swirl it around and smell it before you add the next essential oil.

a) Put 1 drop of ylang ylang essential oil in a dark bottle, swirl and sniff

b) Add 2 drops of lavender essential oil, swirl and sniff

c) Add 3 drops of orange essential oil, swirl and sniff

6. After getting a scent that pleases you, you can now add the essential oils blend to the other natural perfume ingredients.

***

Practical Example 4 of Blending Essential Oils

1. Decide what condition you want your essential oil blend to manage.

Anxiety

2. Choose approximately three essential oils that can manage that condition.

Essential oils that are used to relieve anxiety include bergamot, clary sage, Roman chamomile, geranium, lavender, rose, sandalwood and ylang ylang essential oil.

Chosen essential oils: Lavender essential oil, clary sage essential oil and ylang ylang essential oil

3. Divide those essential oils into top notes, middle notes and base notes.

Top note: clary sage, Middle note: lavender, Base note: ylang ylang

4. Blend your essential oils by adding 1 drop of the base note for every 2 drops of the middle note and 3 drops of the top note into a dark bottle.

5. Begin by adding the base notes and after adding each essential oil into the bottle, swirl it around and smell it before you add the next essential oil.

a) Put 1 drop of ylang ylang essential oil in a dark bottle, swirl and sniff

b) Add 2 drops of lavender essential oil, swirl and sniff

c) Add 3 drops of clary sage essential oil, swirl and sniff

6. After getting a scent that pleases you, you can now add the essential oils blend to the other natural perfume ingredients.

Practical Example 5 of Blending Essential Oils

1. Decide what condition you want your perfume essential oil blend to manage.

Poor concentration

2. Choose approximately three essential oils that can manage that condition.

Essential oils that are used to improve mental concentration include peppermint, eucalyptus, lemon and rosemary essential oils.

Chosen essential oils: Eucalyptus essential oil, lemon essential oil and peppermint essential oil

3. Divide those essential oils into top notes, middle notes and base notes.

Top notes: eucalyptus and lemon, Middle note: peppermint

4. Blend your essential oils by adding 1 drop of the base note for every 2 drops of the middle note and 3 drops of the top note into a dark bottle.

5. Begin by adding the base notes and after adding each essential oil into the bottle, swirl it around and smell it before you add the next essential oil.

a) Add 2 drops of peppermint essential oil in a dark bottle, swirl and sniff

b) Add 3 drops of eucalyptus essential oil and 3 drops of lemon essential oil, swirl and sniff

6. After getting a scent that pleases you, add the essential oil blend to the other natural perfume ingredients.

***

Practical Example 6 of Blending Essential Oils

1. Decide what condition you want your perfume essential oil blend to manage.

Sleeplessness or insomnia

2. Choose approximately three essential oils that can manage that condition.

Essential oils that are used to manage insomnia include lavender, Roman chamomile and ylang ylang essential oils.

Chosen essential oils: Roman chamomile essential oil, clary sage essential oil and ylang ylang essential oil

3. Divide those essential oils into top notes, middle notes and base notes.

Top notes: clary sage, Middle note: roman chamomile, Base note: ylang ylang

4. Blend your essential oils by adding 1 drop of the base note for every 2 drops of the middle note and 3 drops of the top note into a dark bottle.

5. Begin by adding the base notes and after adding each essential oil into the bottle, swirl it around and smell it before you add the next essential oil.

a) Put 1 drop of ylang ylang essential oil in a dark bottle, swirl and sniff

b) Add 2 drops of roman chamomile essential oil, swirl and sniff

c) Add 3 drops of clary sage essential oil, swirl and sniff

6. After getting a scent that pleases you, add the essential oil blend to the other natural perfume ingredients.

***

Practical Example 7 of Blending Essential Oils

1. Decide what condition you want your essential oil blend to manage.

Impotence and frigidity

2. Choose approximately three essential oils that can manage that condition.

Essential oils that are used as aphrodisiacs include bergamot, clary sage, lavender, peppermint, cedarwood, clove, ginger, jasmine, neroli, patchouli, rose, vanilla and ylang ylang essential oil.

Chosen essential oils: Lavender essential oil, clary sage essential oil and ylang ylang essential oil

3. Divide those essential oils into top notes, middle notes and base notes.

Top note: clary sage, Middle note: lavender, Base note: ylang ylang and rose

4. Blend your essential oils by adding 1 drop of the base note for every 2 drops of the middle note and 3 drops of the top note into a dark bottle.

5. Begin by adding the base notes and after adding each essential oil into the bottle, swirl it around and smell it before you add the next essential oil.

a) Put 1 drop of ylang ylang essential oil and 1 drop of rose in a dark bottle, swirl and sniff

b) Add 2 drops of lavender essential oil, swirl and sniff

c) Add 3 drops of clary sage essential oil, swirl and sniff

6. After getting a scent that pleases you or the total number of drops that you need for your recipe, you can now add the blended essential oils to the other ingredients of your recipe.

Practical Example 8 of Blending Essential Oils

1. Decide what condition you want your perfume essential oil blend to manage.

Menopause

2. Choose approximately three essential oils that can manage that condition.

Essential oils used to manage menopausal symptoms include clary sage, geranium, lavender, peppermint, Roman chamomile, and rosemary essential oils.

Chosen essential oils: Lavender essential oil, clary sage essential oil and geranium essential oil

3. Divide those essential oils into top notes, middle notes and base notes.

Top note: clary sage, Middle note: lavender, geranium

4. Blend your essential oils by adding 1 drop of the base note for every 2 drops of the middle note and 3 drops of the top note into a dark bottle.

5. Begin by adding the base notes and after adding each essential oil into the bottle, swirl it around and smell it before you add the next essential oil.

a) Put 2 drops of geranium essential oil and 2 drops of lavender essential oil in a dark bottle, swirl and sniff

b) Add 3 drops of clary sage essential oil, swirl and sniff

6. After getting a scent that pleases you, add the essential oil blend to the other natural perfume ingredients.

***

Practical Example 9 of Blending Essential Oils

1. Decide what condition you want your perfume essential oil blend to manage.

Premenstrual tension (PMS)

2. Choose approximately three essential oils that can manage that condition.

Essential oils used to manage menstrual symptoms include clary sage, geranium, lavender and Roman chamomile essential oils.

Chosen essential oils: Lavender essential oil, clary sage essential oil and ylang ylang essential oil

3. Divide those essential oils into top notes, middle notes and base notes.

Top note: clary sage, Middle note: lavender, Base note: ylang ylang

4. Blend your essential oils by adding 1 drop of the base note for every 2 drops of the middle note and 3 drops of the top note into a dark bottle.

5. Begin by adding the base notes and after adding each essential oil into the bottle, swirl it around and smell it before you add the next essential oil.

a) Put 1 drop of ylang ylang and 2 drops of geranium essential oil in a dark bottle, swirl and sniff

b) Add 3 drops of clary sage essential oil, swirl and sniff

6. After getting a scent that pleases you, add the essential oil blend to the other natural perfume ingredients.

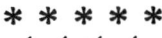

2

CARRIER OILS

Fractionated coconut oil is the best carrier oil for making liquid perfumes because it is odorless and colorless and it can be sprayed through a pump sprayer because of its thin viscosity. Jojoba can also be used to make liquid perfumes.

Virgin coconut oil and olive oil are carrier oils which are used for making solid natural perfumes.

Fractionated Coconut Oil

Botanical name: Cocos nucifera

Also known as FCO or light coconut oil

It is made from virgin coconut oil which undergoes a physical separation process to leave only the medium chain triglycerides in the oil so that it will remain liquid at room temperature.

It is odorless and colorless and it can be sprayed through a pump sprayer because of its thin viscosity.

It is highly stable and has a very long shelf life and is also one of the least expensive carrier oils.

It is readily absorbed as it penetrates the skin well since it has a similar molecular structure to the skin's natural sebum. It also softens and moisturizes the skin

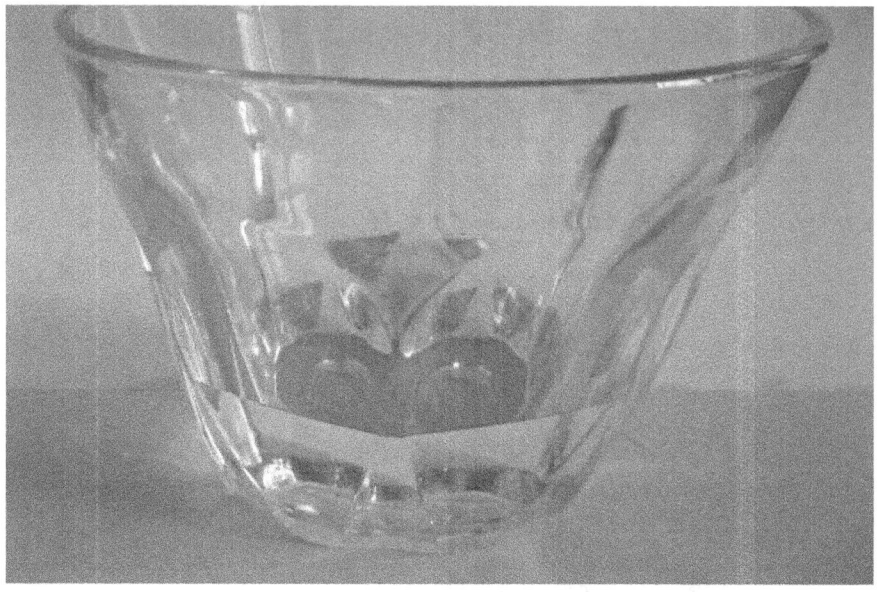

***

Jojoba

Botanical name: Simmondsia chinensis

It is a liquid plant wax and not a vegetable oil.

Its chemical composition is similar to that of the skin's own sebum or oil.

It has natural sunscreens and a SPF of 4

It has a very long shelf life since it is highly stable, has a waxy nature and antibacterial properties.

It contains vitamin E, proteins, minerals, skin nourishing fatty acids and protective antioxidants.

It has a pleasant aroma.

It is moderately light and has a medium viscosity.

It is readily absorbed by the skin resulting in a non-oily softening effect.

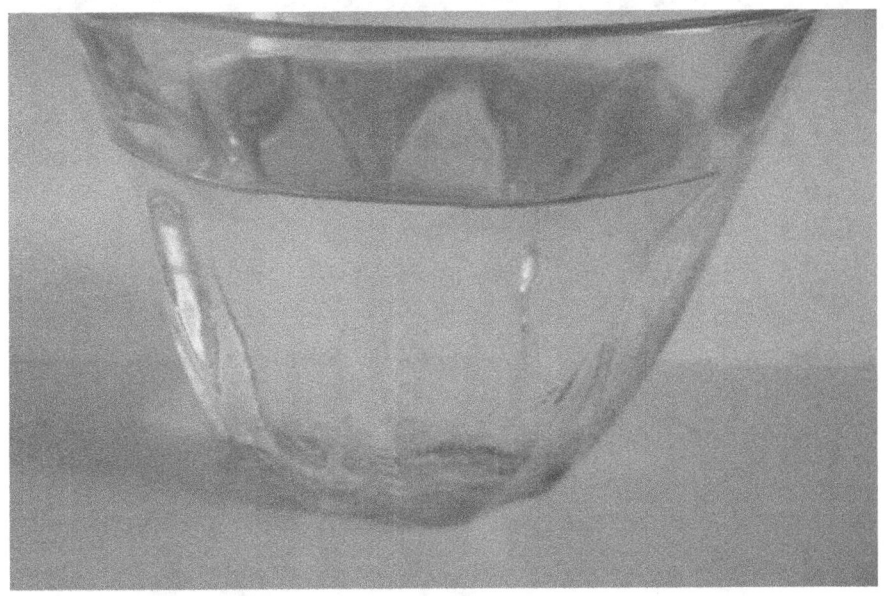

***

Olive Oil

Botanical name: Olea europaea

It has a cooking olive oil aroma.

It has a thick viscosity.

It contains vitamins, skin nourishing essential fatty acids

It has natural sunscreens and a SPF of 2-8

It has a thick viscosity.

It softens and moisturizes the skin.

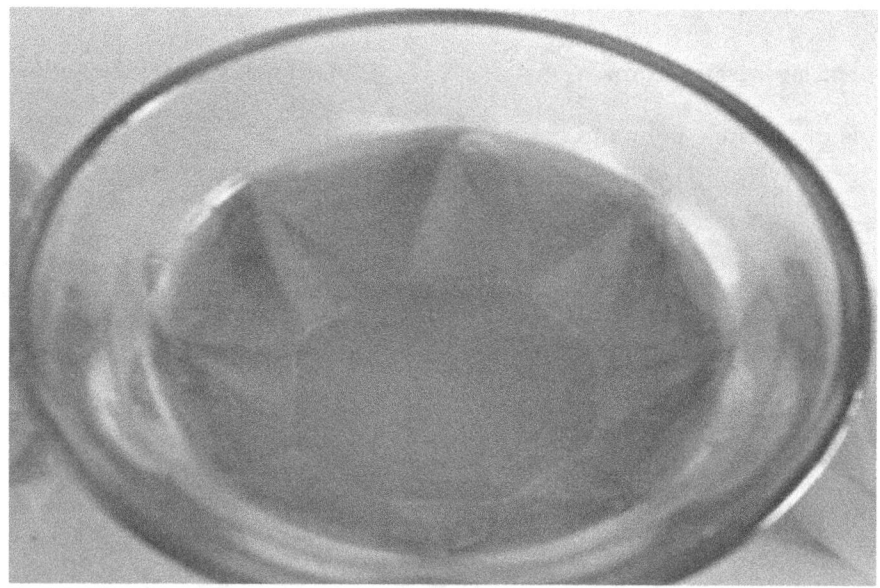

***

Virgin Coconut Oil

Botanical name: Cocos nucifera

It has a fragrant coconut aroma

It is solid at room temperature and melts at 76 degrees.

It contains skin and hair nourishing fatty acids.

It has an estimated SPF of 4-10

It softens and moisturizes the skin.

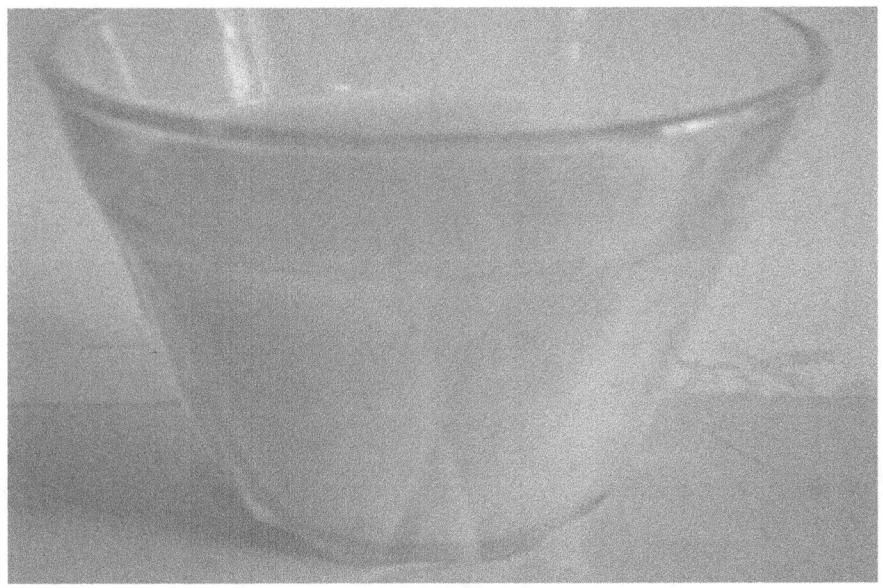

* * * * *

3

AROMATIC CONCENTRATION

In general, when making perfumes, essential oils should be diluted with carrier oils to attain a 3% concentration. This is not a fixed figure and you can make perfumes that are more or less concentrated.

1% concentration

1% concentration = 1 drop of essential oil mixed with 0.17 fl. Oz or 5 ml (1 teaspoon) of carrier oil

1% concentration = 7 drops of essential oil mixed with 1 fl. Oz or 30 ml of carrier oil.

This 1% concentration is generally used on the face, by children and the elderly.

Therefore, if your blended essential oils mixture contains a total of 7 drops of the different essential oils you have used, to create a perfume with a 1% concentration, add the 7 drops of the essential oil blend to 1 fl. Oz or 30 ml of your carrier oil.

***

2% concentration

2% concentration = 2 drops of essential oil mixed with 0.17 fl. Oz or 5 ml (1 teaspoon) of carrier oil

2% concentration = 14 drops of essential oil mixed with 2 fl. Oz or 60 ml of carrier oil.

Therefore, if your blended essential oils mixture contains a total of 7 drops of the different essential oils you have used, to create a perfume with a 2% concentration, add the 7 drops of the essential oil blend to ½ fl. Oz or 15 ml of your carrier oil.

***

3% concentration

3% concentration = 3 drops of essential oil mixed with 0.17 fl. Oz or 5 ml (1 teaspoon) of carrier oil

3% concentration = 21 drops of essential oil mixed with 1 fl. Oz or 90 ml of carrier oil.

This 3% concentration is generally used on the rest of the body.

Therefore, if your blended essential oils mixture contains a total of 7 drops of the different essential oils you have used, to create a perfume with a 3% concentration that can be used on the body, add the 7 drops of the essential oil blend to 1/3 fl. Oz or 10 ml of your carrier oil.

* * * * *

4

HOW TO MAKE LIQUID PERFUMES

There following are three methods for making liquid perfumes with your essential oil blend.

Method A

Ingredients

Essential oil blend 7 drops

Fractionated coconut oil 1/3 fl. oz or 10 ml

Equipment

Dark bottle with a pump sprayer

Droppers

Notebook and pen to jot down your recipe so that you can recreate it if you like it

Instructions

1. Mix the essential oils and the carrier oil in a dark bottle with a pump sprayer. This will create a perfume with a 3% concentration.

2. Keep the bottle in a cool, dark place for 2 days to 2 months to let the perfume mature keeping in mind that the longer it stands, the stronger it will be.

***

Method B

Ingredients

Essential oil blend 7 drops

Fractionated coconut oil or jojoba 1/6 fl. oz or 5 ml

99% alcohol isopropyl 5 ml

Distilled water (optional)

Equipment

Dark bottle with a pump sprayer

Droppers

Notebook and pen to jot down your recipe so that you can recreate it if you like it

Instructions

1. Mix the blended essential oils with the jojoba or fractionated coconut oil in a dark bottle with a pump spray.

2. Add the 99% alcohol isopropyl

3. Keep the bottle in a cool, dark place for 2 days to 2 months to let the perfume mature keeping in mind that the longer it stands, the stronger it will be.

4. If the perfume is too strong for you after it has matured, you can add some distilled water to dilute it.

***

Method C

Ingredients

Essential oil blend 10 ml

99% alcohol isopropyl 37.5 ml

Distilled water 2.5 ml

Equipment

Dark bottle with a pump sprayer

Droppers

Notebook and pen to jot down your recipe so that you can recreate it if you like it

Instructions

1. Mix the essential oils and the carrier oil and the alcohol in a dark bottle with a pump sprayer.

2. Keep the bottle in a cool, dark place for 2 days to 2 months to let the perfume mature keeping in mind that the longer it stands, the stronger it will be.

* * * * *

5

NATURAL LIQUID PERFUME RECIPE TIPS

1. You can use herb infused vegetable oils to give your all natural perfumes subtle scent and color.

For example you can infuse the fractionated coconut oil with rose petals by adding the dry rose petals and leaving it in a bright sunny place for two to six weeks as you shake it daily. Use this rose infused oil to dilute the essential oils and make your liquid perfume.

You can also add lavender flower heads to the carrier oils and thus create oils with the delicate and relaxing lavender scent.

Rosemary infused vegetable oils create a stimulating, greenish oil.

2. You can choose to create a single note fragrance by just using one essential oil in your natural perfume recipe.

***

3. You can also choose to blend the essential oils according to their scent families: for example you can use:

Fresh scents like lemon, orange, bergamot, grapefruit.

Floral scents like rose, lavender, geranium.

Oriental scents like vanilla, clove.

Woody scents like sandalwood, cedar.

* * * * *

6

HOW TO MAKE SOLID PERFUMES

Ingredients

Essential oil blend 14 drops

Carrier oils like fractionated coconut oil or jojoba 2 teaspoons or 10 ml

Grated beeswax 2 teaspoons or 10 ml

Equipment

Small jars or lip balm tubes or old lockets

Droppers

Notebook and pen to jot down your recipe so that you can recreate it if you like it

Instructions

1. Melt the beeswax and carrier oils over a double boiler.

2. Once the beeswax melts remove from the heat source and allow to cool.

3. Add the essential oils as you stir.

4. Pour mixture into your containers and allow it to set.

7

ESSENTIAL OILS

Choose the aromatherapy essential oils you will use for your all natural perfume depending on the effect you want it to have.

Clary Sage Essential Oil has an herbaceous scent. It can help relieve stress related tension, reduce irritability and help one relax. It is also used for the management of mature and acne prone skin. Do not use it during pregnancy or if you are drinking alcohol or driving or if you have endometriosis, ovarian cysts, uterine cysts, breast cancer or you are at high risk for developing breast cancer as it may have an "estrogen-like" effect on the body.

Eucalyptus essential oil has an invigorating scent. It can help relieve stress related mental tension and mental exhaustion. It is also used in the management of joint aches and pains. Do not use it if you have epilepsy, high blood pressure or apply it near a baby's nostrils.

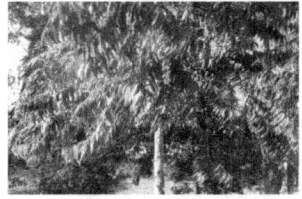

Geranium Essential Oil has a fresh, minty rose scent. It can help relieve nervous tension and anxiety. It is also used in the management of eczema, cellulite as well as mature skin. Avoid using it in pregnancy.

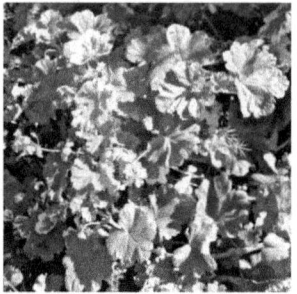

Grapefruit essential oil has a refreshing, bitter-sweet scent. It can help relieve tension and release repressed emotions. It is also used in the management of cellulite.

Lavender essential oil has a soothing, floral scent. It can help one relax and relieve stress related tension, sleeplessness, anxiety and depression. It is also used in the management of acne, eczema and dry skin conditions. Do not use lavender essential oil in pregnancy, if you are breastfeeding, on young children as it may cause breast development in young boys and girls. Avoid it if you have low blood pressure as you may feel drowsy after using it.

Lemon essential oil has an clarifying fresh scent. It can help relieve mental tension, alleviate mental fatigue and increase concentration. It is also used in the management of acne and post acne dark skin spots. Do not use it if skin will be exposed to sunlight or UV rays in the next 12-24 hours. Do not use it if you have low blood pressure or you are allergic to lemons.

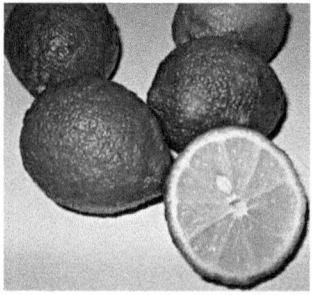

Lemongrass essential oil has a vitalizing, lemony scent. It can help relieve tension and muscle aches. It is also used in the management of acne. Do not use it if skin will be exposed to sunlight or UV rays in the next 12-24 hours.

Roman chamomile essential oil has a sweet and fruity scent. It can help relieve stress related tension headaches. It is also used in the management of eczema, psoriasis and dry skin conditions. Avoid using it in pregnancy and if you are allergic to ragweed.

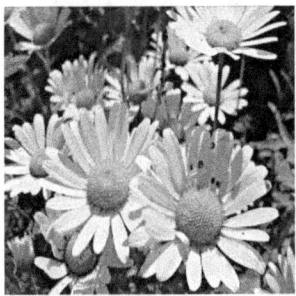

Spearmint essential oil has a gently-energizing minty scent. It can help relieve mental tension and exhaustion. It is also used in the management of nausea.

Rose essential oil has a sweet and floral scent. It has mentally cheering properties and is used to relieve depression, sorrow and heartache. It is also useful for mature and prematurely aging skin.

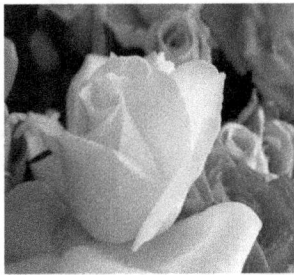

Rosemary Essential Oil has an uplifting and stimulating scent. It can help relieve mental exhaustion and feeling rundown. It is also used in the management of eczema, muscle aches and joint pains. Do not use rosemary essential oil if you are pregnant or have epilepsy or high blood pressure. Avoid using it if you have a fever or you want to sleep and in children under 5 years.

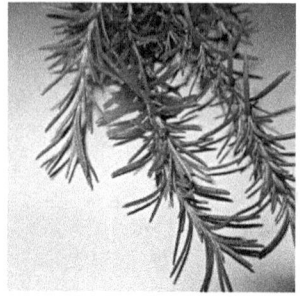

Sweet orange essential oil has a cheeringly, refreshing scent. It can help mange stress related tension. It is also used in the management of cellulite and common colds. Do not use it if skin will be exposed to sunlight or UV rays in the next 12-24 hours.

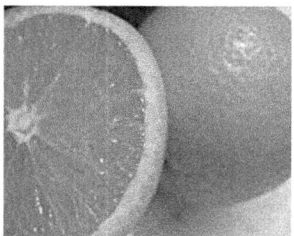

Peppermint essential oil has a head-clearing, refreshing scent. It can help relieve tension and fatigue. It is also used to manage flatulence. Do not use peppermint essential oil in pregnancy, if breastfeeding, on children less than 5 years, if you have epilepsy or irregular heart beats or cardiac fibrillation or high blood pressure and before using a sun bed or going to hot humid places.

Tea tree essential oil has a purifying almost medicinal scent. It can help relieve tension and fatigue. It is also been used in the management of acne and athlete's foot.

Ylang ylang Essential Oil has a fragrantly floral scent. It can help relieve anxiety, tension and help one relax. It is also used as an aphrodisiac and in the management of dry skin conditions. Do not use ylang ylang essential oil if you have low blood pressure or sensitive, damaged skin.

###

ABOUT THE AUTHOR

Dr. Miriam Kinai is a medical doctor and a certified clinical aromatherapy practitioner.

You can visit her blog at http://thetoparomatherapysite.blogspot.com/ or follow her on twitter at http://twitter.com/AlmasiHealth

Email enquiries to almasihealthcare@yahoo.com with BOOKS as your subject.

HOW TO MAKE NATURAL SKIN CARE PRODUCTS VOLUME 1

How To Make Natural Skin Care Products Volume 1 by Dr Miriam Kinai is filled with recipes for making organic bath and body products for normal, sensitive, oily and dry skin types as well as therapeutic products to manage mature skin, prematurely aging skin, cellulite, eczema, psoriasis, ringworms, dandruff, thinning hair, menopausal symptoms, pre-menstrual tension (PMS), painful periods, arthritis, stress, sadness or depression, mental exhaustion and insomnia.

This book also teaches you the best vegetable oils, essential oils, natural butters and herbs to use when making products for different skin types physical conditions. You will learn how to make:

* Bath bombs

* Bath melts

* Bath salts

* Bath teas

* Body butters

* Body lotions

* Body scrubs

* Healing balms and body creams

* Herb infused oils

* Natural soap

How to Make Natural Skin Care Products Volume 1 will leave you with a clear understanding of how to make bath and beauty products to use in your home or to give as gifts or to sell and make money.

*****

THE ESSENTIALS OF AROMATHERAPY ESSENTIAL OILS

The Essentials of Aromatherapy Essential Oils by Dr Miriam Kinai teaches you how to use aromatherapy oils to improve your physical, mental and emotional well being.

The author's experience as a medical doctor and clinical aromatherapy practitioner have enabled her to write a highly informative guide for those who want to utilize the healing benefits of these natural plant essences.

You will discover:

* The safety information and therapeutic uses of 18 essential oils

* How to blend essential oils

* The characteristics and uses of 14 carrier oils

* How to Dilute Essential Oils with Carrier Oils

* How to Use Essential Oils

* Cautionary Measures when using Essential Oils

* Numerous Essential Oil Recipes for bath products as well as skin care and hair care products

The Essentials of Aromatherapy Essential Oils will leave you with a clear understanding of how you can safely use aromatherapy essential oils to heal yourself naturally.

*****

MEDICAL AROMATHERAPY FOR HEALTH PROFESSIONALS

Medical Aromatherapy for Healthcare Professionals by Dr Miriam Kinai teaches you how to use essential oils to treat physical diseases and emotional disorders.

The author's experience as a medical doctor and clinical aromatherapy practitioner have enabled her to write a highly informative guide for those who want to utilize the healing benefits of these natural plant essences.

You will discover how to use essential oils to:

* Treat skin diseases like acne, eczema and psoriasis

* Treat other physical diseases like high blood pressure, arthritis, coughs and colds

* Manage mental and emotional conditions like anxiety, depression, anger and stress

* Relieve the symptoms of menopause and premenstrual tension

* Lessen insomnia and impotence

Medical Aromatherapy for Healthcare Professionals is therefore an essential resource for holistic healthcare practitioners like massage therapists, naturopaths and herbalists.

It is also a useful resource for conventional medicine healthcare providers like physicians and nurses who want to begin practicing integrative medicine and for patients who want to improve their health naturally by using aromatherapy oils.

*****

AROMATHERAPY COURSE

Aromatherapy Course by Dr Miriam Kinai tutors you on how to use essential oils to improve your physical, mental and emotional well being.

The author's experience as a medical doctor and clinical aromatherapy practitioner have enabled her to create a highly informative course on how to use these natural plant essences.

You will learn:

* The safety information and therapeutic uses of essential oils like clary sage, eucalyptus, geranium, grapefruit, lavender, lemon, lemongrass, marjoram, orange (sweet), patchouli, peppermint, Roman chamomile, rose, rosemary, sandalwood, spearmint, tea tree and ylang ylang.

* The safety information and therapeutic uses of carrier oils like apricot kernel oil, avocado oil, borage seed oil, calendula oil, carrot seed oil, castor oil, evening primrose oil, fractionated coconut oil, jojoba, olive oil, rosehip oil, sunflower oil, sweet almond oil and virgin coconut oil.

* How to blend essential oils

* How to dilute essential oils with carrier oils

* How to administer essential oils

* How to make natural healing products from numerous aromatherapy recipes

* How to utilize the healing benefits of essentials oils even if you do not have prior training in aromatherapy

The Aromatherapy Course will leave you with a clear understanding of how you can heal yourself and your family naturally by using essentials oils on your body and in your home.

*****

DARK SKIN DERMATOLOGY COLOR ATLAS

Dark Skin Dermatology Color Atlas is filled with clear explanations and color photos of skin, hair, and nail diseases affecting people with skin of color or Fitzpatrick skin types IV, V, and VI.

Topics covered include Acne Vulgaris, Alopecia Areata, Anal Warts, Angioedema, Aphthous Ulcers, Atopic Dermatitis, Blastomycosis, Blister Beetle Dermatitis or Nairobi Fly Dermatitis, Cellulitis, Chronic Ulcers, Confetti Hypopigmentation, Cutaneous T Cell Lymphoma, Cutaneous Tuberculosis, Dermatitis Artefacta, Erythema Nodosum,

Exfoliative Erythroderma, Gianotti Crosti Syndrome, Hand Dermatitis, Hemangioma, Herpes Zoster, Ichthyosis, Ingrown Toenails, Irritant Contact Dermatitis, Kaposi Sarcoma, Keloids, Keratoderma Blenorrhagica, Klippel Trenaunay Weber Syndrome, Leishmaniasis, Leprosy, Leukonychia, Lichen Nitidus, Lichen Planus,

Lichenoid Drug Eruption, Linear Epidermal Nevus, Linear IgA Dermatosis (LAD), Lipodermatosclerosis, Lymphangioma Circumscriptum, Miliaria, Molluscum Contagiosum, Neurofibromatosis, Nickel Dermatitis, Onychomadesis, Onychomycosis, Palmoplantar Eccrine Hidradenitis, Papular Pruritic Eruption (PPE), Paronychia, Pellagra, Pemphigus Foliaceous,

Pemphigus Vulgaris, Piebaldism, Pityriasis Rosea, Pityriasis Rubra Pilaris, Plantar Hyperkeratosis, Plantar Warts, Poikiloderma, Postinflammatory Hyperpigmentation and Hypopigmentation, Post Topical Steroids Hypopigmentation, Psoriasis, Pyogenic Granuloma or Lobular Capillary Hemangioma, Scabies, Seborrheic Dermatitis, Steven Johnson Syndrome (SJS) and Toxic Epidermal Necrolysis (TEN),

Sunburn, Systemic Sclerosis, Tinea Capitis, Tinea Pedis, Tinea Versicolor, Traction Alopecia, Urticaria, Vasculitis, Vitiligo, and Xanthelasma.

*****